Sjögren's Syndrome
in Clinical Practice

Graham Hughes • Shirish Sangle
Simon Bowman

Sjögren's Syndrome in Clinical Practice

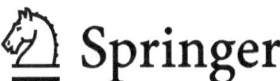 Springer

Graham Hughes
The London Lupus Centre
London Bridge Hospital
London
United Kingdom

Shirish Sangle
Louise Coote Lupus Unit
St Thomas' Hospital
London
United Kingdom

Simon Bowman
Department of Rheumatology
Queen Elizabeth Medical
Centre
Birmingham
United Kingdom

ISBN 978-3-319-06058-3   ISBN 978-3-319-06059-0   (eBook)
DOI 10.1007/978-3-319-06059-0
Springer Cham Heidelberg New York Dordrecht London

Library of Congress Control Number: 2014940967

Printed on acid-free paper

Springer is part of Springer Science+Business Media (www.springer.com)

Contents

Chapter 1
Introduction

What Is Sjögren's Syndrome?

At its most basic, Sjögren's Syndrome consists of the combination of dry eyes, dry mouth and aches and pains. It is now recognised that the underlying abnormality is a malfunction of the immune system, and that the condition can affect other organs.

It is also recognised now that Sjögren's Syndrome is common and an important cause of aches, pains and fatigue. It is considered by many doctors to be central to the group of so-called 'autoimmune' diseases, overlapping with other important disorders such as Hashimoto's disease (underactive thyroid). Hughes Syndrome (antiphospholipid syndrome) and rheumatoid arthritis (Fig. 1.1).

The dryness of the eyes and of the mouth are caused by inflammation and/or damage to the lachrymal (tear) and salivary glands respectively, the glands being infiltrated by immune 'white' cells (also called 'lymphocytes') that go round the blood stream, lymph nodes, spleen and bone marrow fighting infections such as bacteria or viruses.

Although the precise prevalence is not known, it is estimated that about 1 in a 1,000 to 1 in 200 adult women in the UK have Sjögren's syndrome. It is, however, rare in men with approximately 1 man for every 13 women with the condition (Fig. 1.2). A recent epidemiological study by a French group

G. Hughes et al., *Sjögren's Syndrome in Clinical Practice*,
DOI 10.1007/978-3-319-06059-0_1,
© Springer International Publishing Switzerland 2014

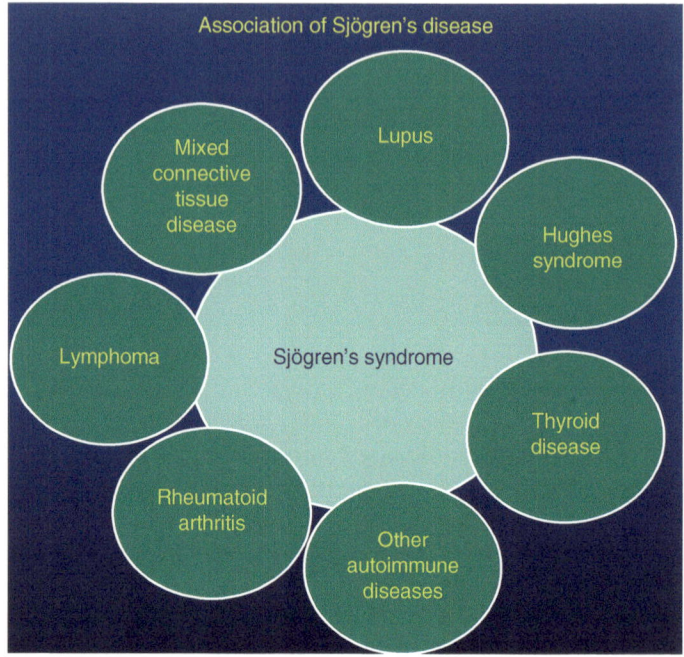

FIGURE 1.1 Association of Sjögren's syndrome with other autoimmune diseases

in a multiethnic population found a prevalence up to 10 per 10,000 population. A genetic predisposition to SS has been suggested. Familial clustering of different autoimmune diseases and co-association of multiple autoimmune diseases in individuals have both frequently been reported. This still makes Sjögren's syndrome one of the most common autoimmune disorders after rheumatoid arthritis, however, this disease is rather under-diagnosed.

History

Early descriptions of the condition were published in 1888 (Hadden), and, in 1892, by Mikulicz who described the case of a German farmer with enlarged parotid glands. The glands

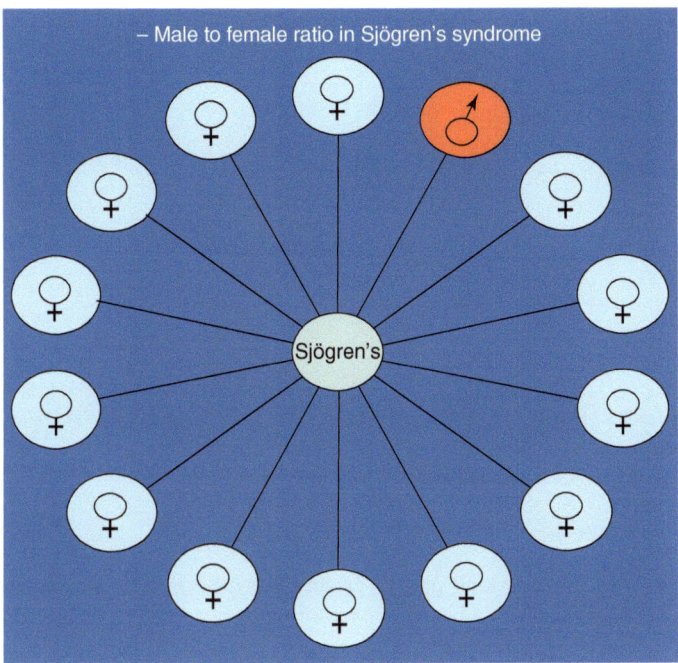

FIGURE 1.2 male to female ration in Sjögren's syndrome

were biopsied and revealed an infiltration of the glandular tissue by lymphocytes.

In 1933, Hendrik Sjögren, a Swedish eye specialist, published a clinical series describing patients with dry eyes, and recognised that more widespread features were also present.

In the 1960s and 1970s, many studies describing auto-antibodies in various diseases were published. Antibodies are small proteins that stick to bacteria or viruses and help clear them from the circulation. We have billions of them in our bloodstream. In autoimmune diseases we often produce antibodies against our own tissues (autoantibodies) that can be identified on blood tests. Two antibodies, so called 'anti-Ro' and 'anti-La' were found to be useful markers for Sjögren's syndrome (Fig. 1.3). In this period, clinical features, laboratory markers and the association with non-Hodgkin's

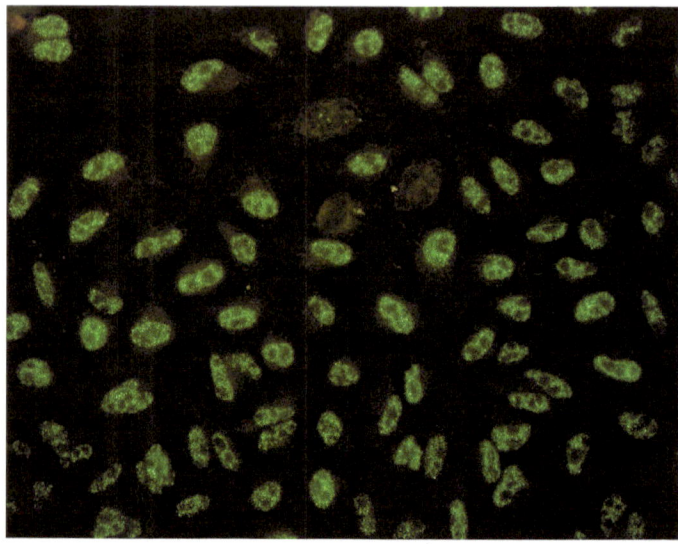

Figure 1.3 Speckled pattern of anti Ro (SSA) antibodies in anti nuclear (ANA) antibody fluorescent test

lymphoma were also identified. In more recent years, a number of studies have focused on genetic and environmental factors in the aetiology of Sjögren's Syndrome. These will be discussed later.

What Are the Symptoms?

The original description of Sjögren's syndrome was limited to dry eyes and mouth due to lack of tears and saliva.

The commonest symptoms are of fatigue and of aches and pains. As tests for rheumatoid arthritis can also be positive in Sjögren's syndrome, patients are often suspected of having 'early' rheumatoid disease, (see Chap. 11). Others may be diagnosed with 'fibromyalgia'. Fatigue is the most commonly observed symptom in Sjögren's occurring up to 70 % of patients. There are no precise markers to measure the fatigue but the negative impact on health can be severe and frequent.

A moderate correlation between depression and fatigue has also been found. One possible explanation is that fatigue and depression share common underlying biological mechanisms.

The dryness of the eyes may be mild – either going unnoticed or causing minor irritation or scratchiness, or can be severe and painful. In other patients, it is the mouth dryness and the difficulty in swallowing dry food which are the more prominent complaints. In some patients, there is intermittent swelling of glands the lymph glands in the neck and/or the salivary glands over the face or beneath the jaw. Very occasionally the parotid glands become so swollen that the patient is wrongly labelled as having mumps.

Although Sjögren's is rarely life threatening (unlike its 'cousin' lupus), it can be a chronic and debilitating condition if left untreated.

Chapter 2
Eyes

The front of the eye and its delicate membrane, the conjunctiva, are kept moist and protected by a thin layer of fluid – tears – secreted by the lachrymal (tear) glands. The disease affects the tear-producing lachrymal glands.

Inflammation of the lachrymal glands interferes with their function and leads to diminished tear secretion. This may lead, in turn, to damage and, in severe cases, destruction of the membrane (the epithelium) of the conjunctiva. Instead of a smooth moist eye surface, the conjunctiva becomes 'scratched' (similar to scratches on one's glasses).

Symptoms

Perhaps the most surprising thing is that some patients with Sjögrens have few symptoms of eye dryness. Some will have noticed a scratching sensation – sometimes itchiness – under the eyelids. Other eye symptoms are grittiness and, occasionally, redness (Fig. 2.1). Gritty eyes symptoms usually develop slowly over a period of several years.

One of the common complaints is of photophobia – an uncomfortable feeling in the eyes, when in bright light. For this reason, it is not surprising that a number of patients with Sjögren's Syndrome find relief with sunglasses.

G. Hughes et al., *Sjögren's Syndrome in Clinical Practice*,
DOI 10.1007/978-3-319-06059-0_2,
© Springer International Publishing Switzerland 2014

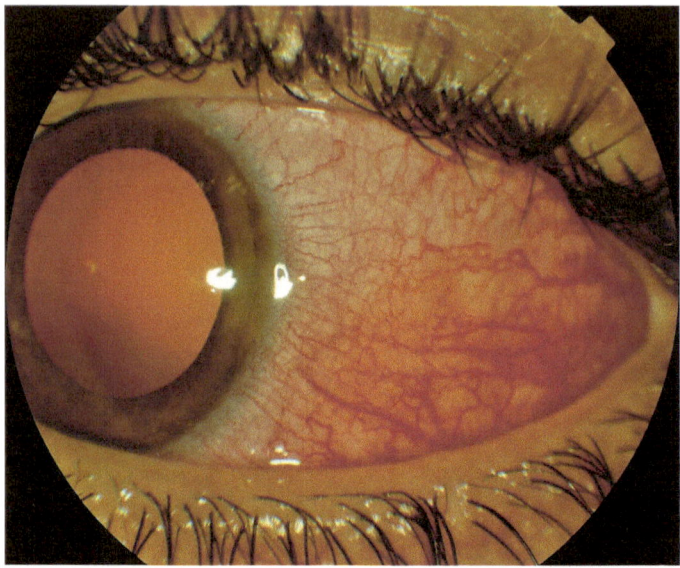

FIGURE 2.1 Dry conjunctiva in Sjogren's syndrome can cause recurrent eye infections

Signs

On casual inspection, there may be no obvious abnormality. Very often, the problem is only recognised when formal testing with blotting paper – the Schirmer's test (see below) – or slit lamp examination (see below), is carried out.

In more severe cases, there may be obvious conjunctiva erosion, or even dilatation of the conjunctiva blood vessels.

In rare cases, the lachrymal glands themselves (situated in the upper, outside corner of the eye orbit) may be enlarged.

Some patients have irritation and redness of the eyelids (blepharitis) which can be helped by warm compresses and careful eyelid hygiene.

Tests for Eye Involvement

Schirmer's Test

This simple 'filter paper' test is a very useful diagnostic aid. Strips of standardised filter paper are hooked over the lower eyelid (Fig. 2.2). After 5 min the length of wetted blotting paper is recorded. In a normal eye, wetting is immediate (and usually copious). In Sjögren's Syndrome there is little wetting (Less than or equal to 5 mm in 5 min is taken as 'dry').

Slit Lamp Examination (Fig. 2.3)

Rose bengal is a dye which has the property of staining damaged epithelium, picking up lesions both in the cornea and in the conjunctiva. A dry eye with an inadequate tear film will show areas of damage and these areas of damage, stained by the Rose Bengal dye are visualised by routine slit-lamp examination.

Rose Bengal dye is quite irritating to the eyes and in many departments has been replaced by a green dye – lissamine green, which is used in a similar way.

Another helpful part of the slit-lamp examination is to use fluorescein dye to stain the tears and ask the patient to blink thus spreading the tears across the eyes. Counting the time that it takes for the tear film to break up after re-opening the eyes (the tear film break up time), this gives an indication of the amount of tears – the shorter the break-up time the fewer the tears and the dryer the eye.

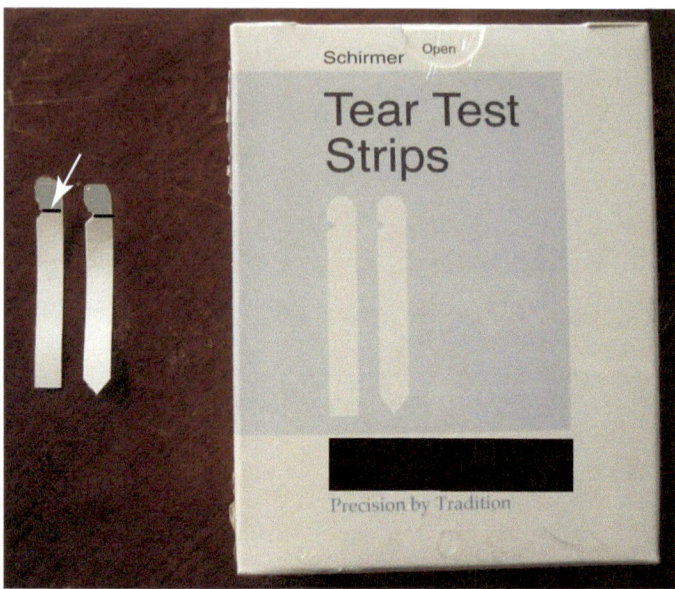

FIGURE 2.2 Dry Schirmer's test showing reduced lachrymal secretion

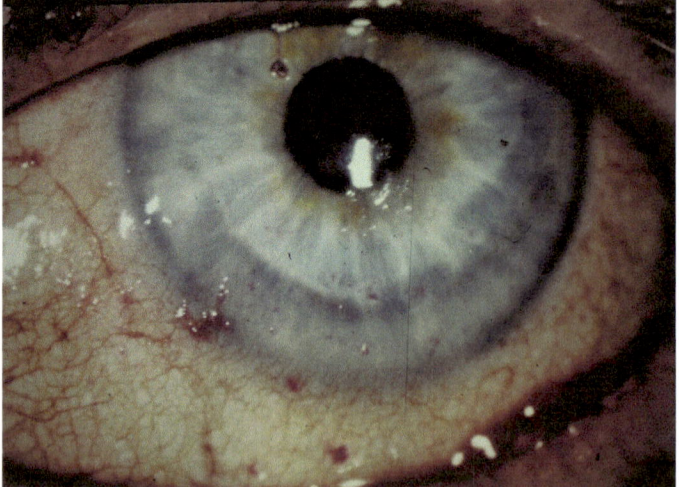

FIGURE 2.3 Rose bengal test showing damaged conjunctiva due to lack of tears

Chapter 3
Mouth and Salivary Glands

Involvement of the salivary glands (principally the submandibular glands and the parotid glands), leads to poor saliva
output. This in turn leads to a dry mouth – occasionally free
of symptoms, but frequently troublesome (Fig. 3.1).

Dryness in the mouth can sometimes be seen as a lack of
pooling of the saliva under the tongue when the tongue is
held for some moments against the roof of the mouth.

The dryness also affects the tongue, sometimes manifest as
a loss of moisture and even a loss of the normal mucosal cov-
ering of the tongue (Fig. 3.1).

Dryness can also affect swallowing – especially of dry food
such as dry bread or biscuits.

One of the commoner problems for patients with severe
Sjögren's Syndrome is of dental decay. There is an increased
risk of gum resorption and of dental caries and loosening.
Fortunately, the increased recognition of Sjögrens by the dental profession has had a major positive impact in reducing
these complications.

In some patients with Sjögrens (notably in some of those
with primary Sjögrens) (see Chap. 11), there may be prominent swelling of the salivary glands. Usually, the more obviously swollen pair of glands are the parotid glands, sited at
the back of the cheeks just in front of the earlobes. Rarely,
these glands become grossly swollen, (resembling mumps).

Because of the pathology in the glands and the distortion
of the normal anatomy, infection and stone formation are

G. Hughes et al., *Sjögren's Syndrome in Clinical Practice*,
DOI 10.1007/978-3-319-06059-0_3,
© Springer International Publishing Switzerland 2014

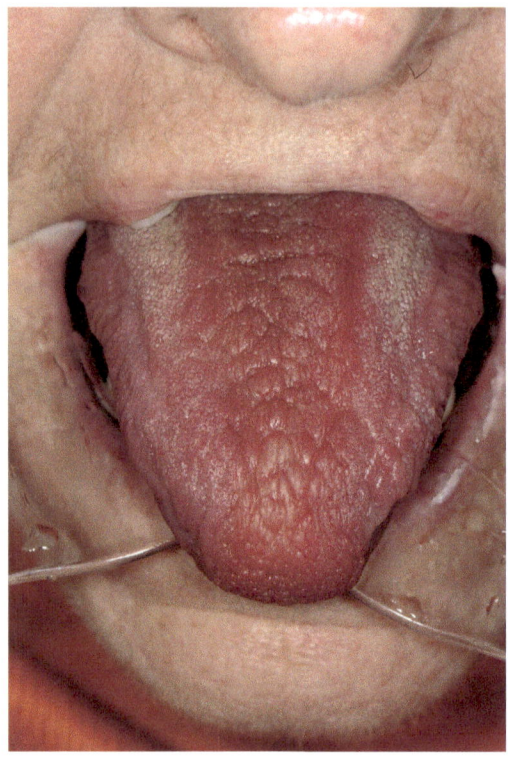

FIGURE 3.1   Dry mouth in Sjögren's syndrome due to lack of salivary secretions

seen in some Sjögren's patients – fortunately a rare phenomenon.

In summary, it is the so-called mucous membranes that are affected in Sjögrens – not only the mouth and the throat, but also the lining of the nose (which can become dry and sore), the vagina and the bladder; but these will be discussed in separate chapters.

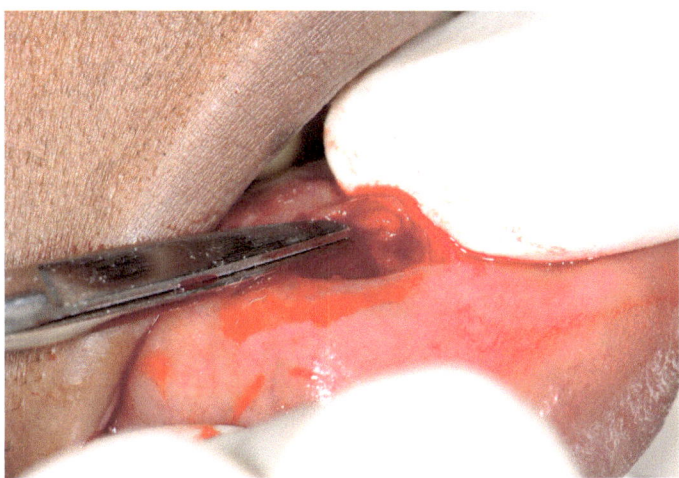

FIGURE 3.2 Lip biopsy for the histopathological diagnosis of Sjögren's syndrome

Diagnosis of the oral manifestations of Sjögren's can involve a lip biopsy (to obtain a 'minor' salivary gland) (Fig. 3.2), sialometry (measurement of salivary flow rates), sialography (a radio contrast examination, especially useful for demonstrating abnormalities in the salivary duct system) and scintigraphy (isotope scanning to demonstrate impaired isotope uptake in Sjögrens). More recently, ultrasound and MRI scanning have also been found to be helpful. These investigations are discussed in more detail in Chap. 14. Since the advent of newer imaging techniques, lip biopsy is not routinely recommended.

Chapter 4
Lungs

The lining of the main breathing tubes – the bronchi – can also be 'dry'. This can lead to a dry cough, in some cases wrongly attributed to asthma.

A more serious (though rare) association is of interstitial lung disease sometimes leading to thickening and scarring of the lungs (pulmonary fibrosis). Interstitial lung disease results from inflammation in the lungs, leading to difficulty in absorbing oxygen into the lungs (Fig. 4.1).

In most cases, the cause is unknown, though in others, there may be a link with work-associated toxins such as silica. The main complaint is of shortness of breath. The lower reaches of the lungs are the most commonly affected. Clinically, listening with a stethoscope can reveal 'scratching' noises in the lower reaches of the lungs, (best heard at the lower back of the chest). One way to think about lung inflammation and fibrosis is to think of the normal lung as candy floss: normally light and airy, but when the edge of the candy floss is licked, the surfaces become matted and less spongy. Other lung manifestations such as inflammation of the lining of the lungs (pleurisy) are more usually seen in those patients with Sjögrens syndrome who have an accompanying 'connective tissue disease', such as rheumatoid arthritis or lupus (see Chap. 11). For the majority of patients with 'primary' Sjögrens, (those cases without an accompanying disease), it should be said that major lung problems are uncommon.

G. Hughes et al., *Sjögren's Syndrome in Clinical Practice*,
DOI 10.1007/978-3-319-06059-0_4,
© Springer International Publishing Switzerland 2014

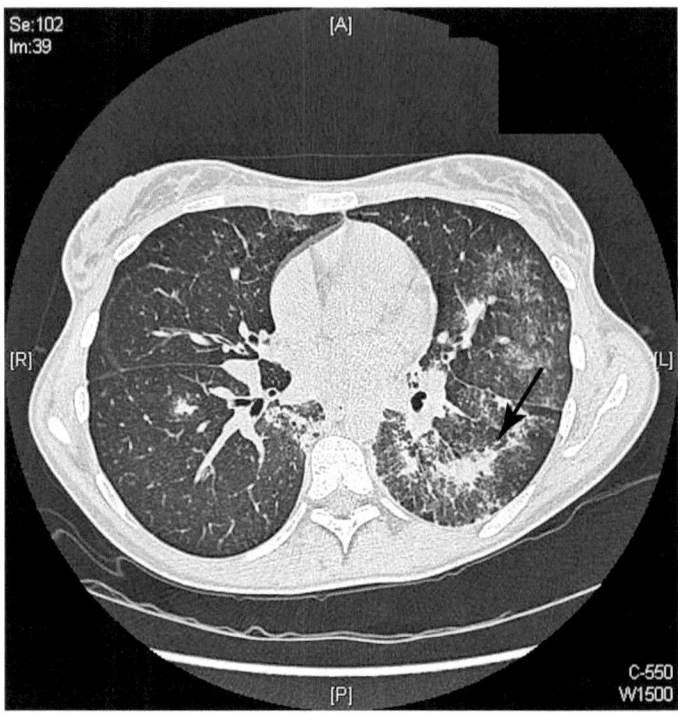

FIGURE 4.1   A CT scan imaging showing intestitial lung disease (lung tissue scarring – pulmonary fibrosis) in Sjogren's syndrome (*arrowed*)

Chapter 5
Skin

Skin involvement is quite common, nearly half of all patients with Sjögren's may present cutaneous manifestations consisting of skin dryness, angular cheilitis, erythema annulare, chilblain lupus and skin vasculitis.

Dryness

Although the main brunt of the 'dryness' in Sjögren's Syndrome falls on 'mucous' surfaces such as the mouth, pharynx, oesophagus, vagina and bladder, the skin can also be affected. Dryness of the skin is often a major complaint in Sjögren's patients. As well as the dryness caused by Sjögren's itself, there are other potential causes – fever, malabsorption, thyroid and other endocrine problems.

Rashes

The skin is sometimes referred to as the 'barometer' of the body. It provides clues to underlying conditions and is an important part of clinical examination. A variety of rashes can be seen in Sjögrens patients. Commonest are allergic rashes. Often itchy and widespread, they can result from allergy to skin contacts, to drugs (especially antibiotics) and

G. Hughes et al., *Sjögren's Syndrome in Clinical Practice*,
DOI 10.1007/978-3-319-06059-0_5,
© Springer International Publishing Switzerland 2014

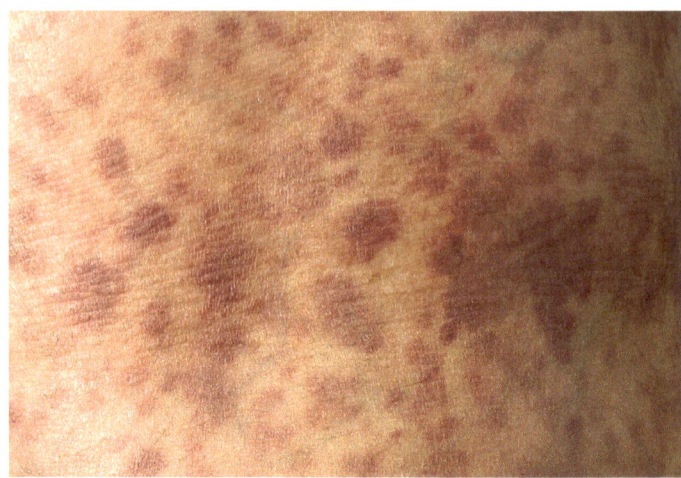

FIGURE 5.1 Urticarial rash seen in Sjögren's syndrome secondary to antibiotics

to food (Fig. 5.1). Some allergies are especially common. One in particular is to the antibiotic 'Septrin' (a sulphur–containing drug rarely used these days). Septrin allergy was so common in both our Sjögrens and our lupus patients that we even include it as a clue when making a diagnosis of these diseases. Other common allergens are sulphonamides and gold salts (once used in the treatment of arthritis).

One interesting allergy is to the antibiotic Minocycline. This drug, widely used for acne, has been implicated in the development of lupus-like features in some patients. It may be that those with underlying Sjögrens are more at risk though this has not been proved as yet.

Raynaud's Phenomenon (Fig. 5.2)

This is a condition in which the fingers can suddenly become white – usually after exposure to cold. After a while, the white turns to blue. When circulation returns, they can become red – white, blue and red!

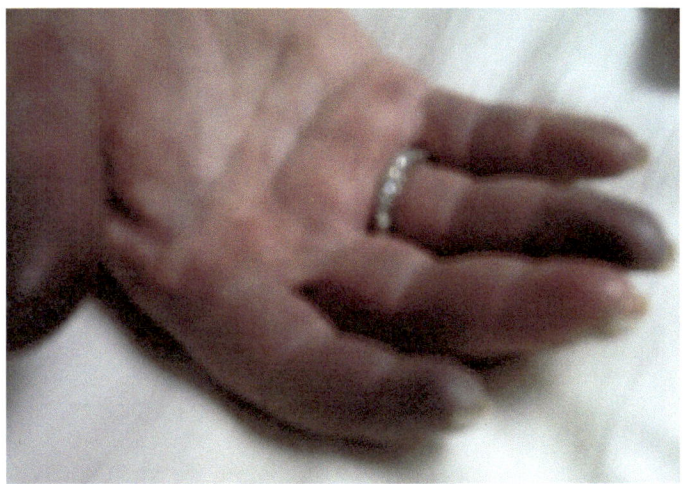

FIGURE 5.2 Raynaud's phenomenon in Sjögren's syndrome

The condition can affect all ten fingers, though sometimes, rather strangely, only one, or two fingers are affected. The toes can also be affected, though less frequently than the fingers.

'Raynauds' is a feature seen in many conditions, though it can also affect healthy people. It is particularly common and severe in scleroderma, and in so-called 'mixed connective tissue disease', and usually milder both in lupus and in Sjögren's Syndrome. Simply wearing warm gloves in the cold is sufficient in most cases. For patients with more severe Raynaud's, medications such as calcium-channel blockers can be helpful.

Sun Sensitivity

A number of Sjögrens patients complain of being sensitive to the sun (or more specifically to UV light).

It can present as a pinkish rash on the cheeks, the eyelids and the v-neck – raising suspicion of the more severe illness

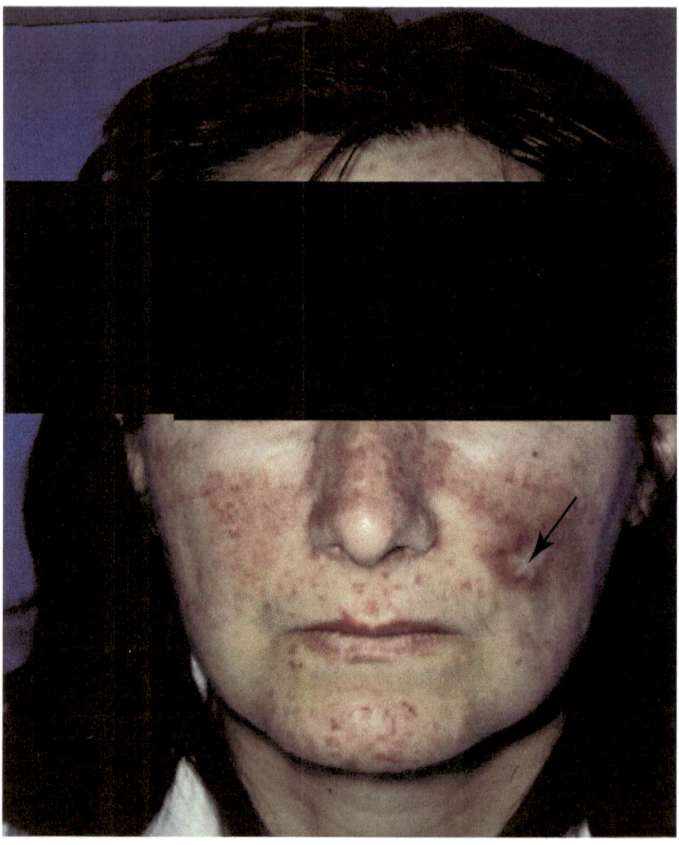

FIGURE 5.3 A photosensitivity butterfly shaped rash and a discoid rash with scarring (see the *arrow*) in a patient with positive anti Ro antibodies

lupus (Fig. 5.3). In most cases, the rashes are mild and transient. A different clinical presentation seen is Sjögren's syndrome is "annular erythema", thought to be highly specific of this syndrome (Fig. 5.4). Since there are common pathophysiologic mechanisms, mainly the presence of anti-Ro/SSA or anti-La/SSB antibodies, it is difficult to separate the annular erythema from subacute cutaneous lupus erythematosus (Fig. 5.5).

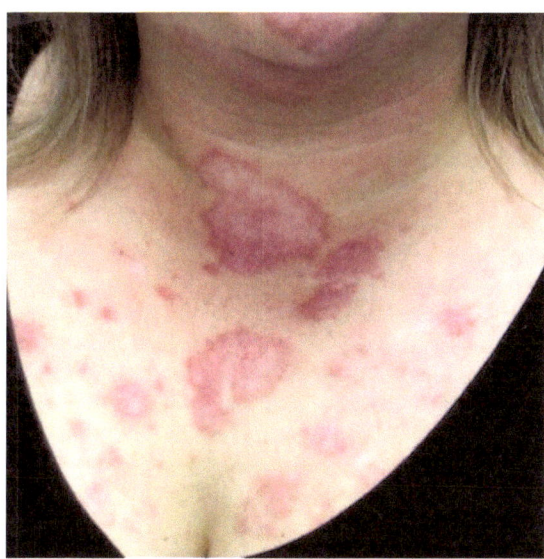

FIGURE 5.4 Subacute cutaneous rash in a patient with positive anti Ro antibodies

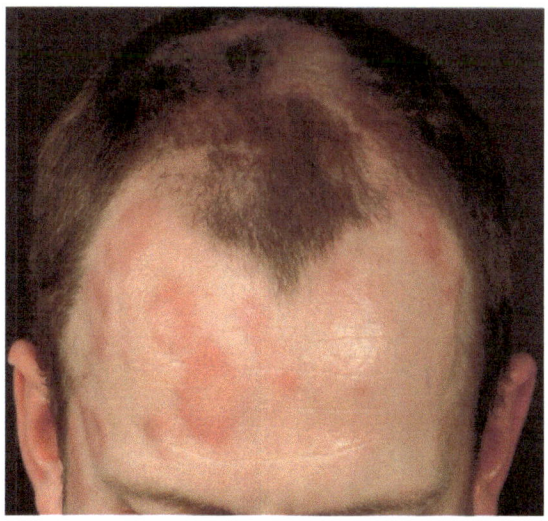

FIGURE 5.5 Subacute cutaneous rash in a male patient with positive anti Ro antibodies

Purpura

Purpura, a collection of small red spots, is seen in some patients with Sjögrens. Classically, it is seen in those with primary Sjögrens (often anti-Ro positive (see page 66).

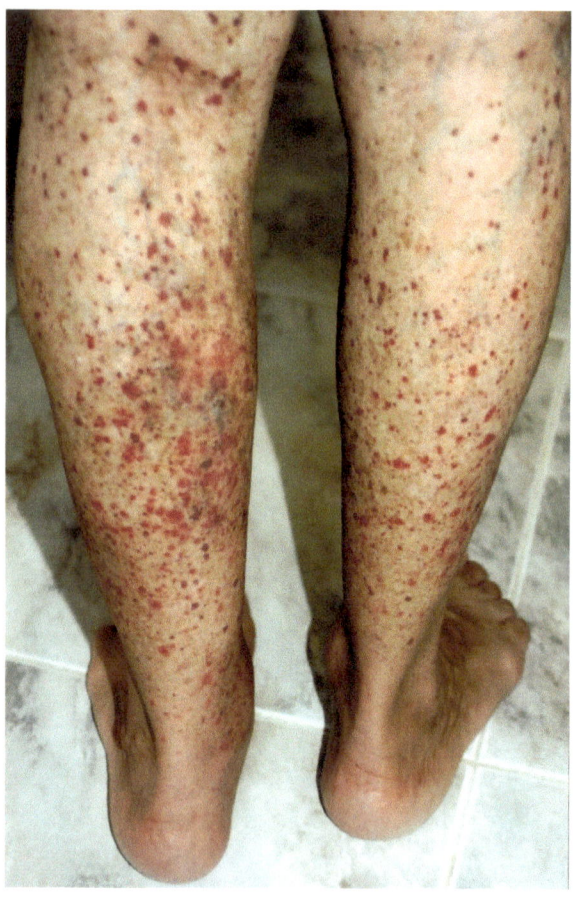

FIGURE 5.6 Purpuric rash on booth legs in a patient with Sjögren's syndrome

It has three main characteristics. Firstly, it usually presents below the knees. Secondly it commonly erupts as a large number (sometimes dozens) of small, (under 1 mm) red spots (Fig. 5.6). Thirdly, it often comes out after exercise or alcohol consumption (Ed Franklin, the New York doctor who made many of the ground-breaking studies of the condition, claimed that most of the cases he had seen followed a game of tennis!). We have also seen the purpuric spots appear in a Sjögren's patient after a long haul flight. These spots are found to be due to a mild inflammation in small blood vessels – so-called vasculitis. The fact that they are often found in those Sjögrens patients with high levels of certain blood proteins (for example: Rheumatoid factor or macro-globulins – see Chap. 14), suggests that blood 'sludging' as well as blood vessel inflammation may also contribute. In a small number of patients, the purpura become chronic, ulti-mately leading to a brownish 'bruised' staining of the shins. Very rarely, the purpura can be spread higher to the thighs and even to the abdomen.

In some patients with purpura, impaired blood supply to the peripheral nerves in the legs (peripheral neuropathy), leads to tingling and numbness in the feet.

Livedo

A blotchy, lacy rash – often on the thighs, the knees and the arms is known as livedo (Fig. 5.7). It is often seen in healthy individuals – women more than men – and is more prominent in the cold. However it can be an important sign of 'auto-immune' diseases – notably Hughes Syndrome. So, in Sjögrens patients, in whom livedo (or livedo reticularis to give it its full name), is found, look for clues to Hughes Syndrome – the antiphospholipid syndrome or 'sticky blood'. These clues can include migraine, memory problems, balance difficulties and angina. More dramatic clues can include a

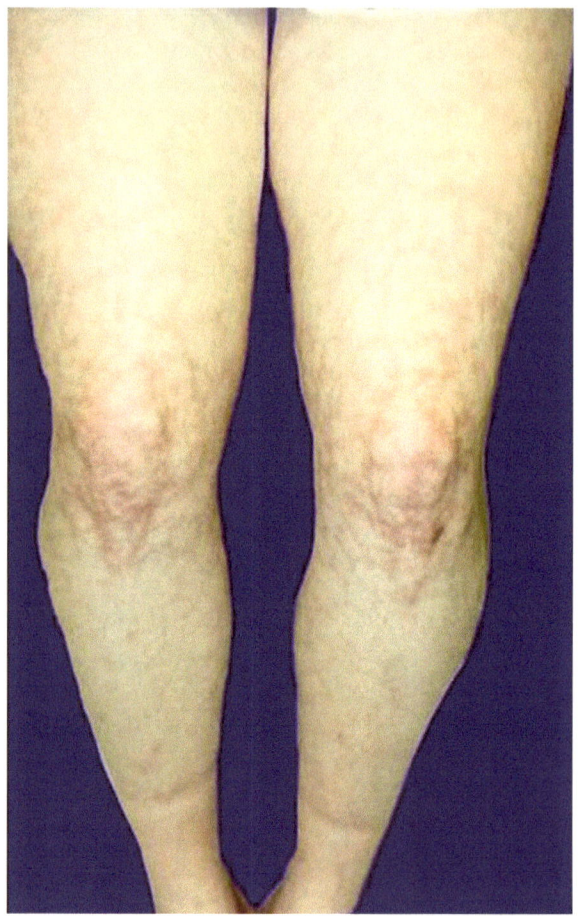

FIGURE 5.7 Livedo reticularis

past history of recurrent miscarriage, a past history of a blood clot or even, in severe cases, symptoms of an early stroke. So, so important, as preventive treatment such as aspirin or even warfarin can be life changing (see Chap. 11)

Neonatal lupus: Mothers with positive anti-Ro antibodies may pass the antibodies through placenta to the infant causing 'target' shaped skin lesions (neonatal lupus) in the new born (see Chap. 11). These rashes are generally self-limiting and disappear within 6 months. This does not mean that the child has lupus or Sjögren's syndrome.

Chapter 6
Gut

Swallowing

The mouth dryness and lack of saliva can lead to difficulties in swallowing – especially of dry food. The dryness can extend down the oesophagus making swallowing even more difficult. Fortunately, in Sjögren's syndrome, this rarely produces major difficulties, though in a number of the other connective tissue diseases such as scleroderma, food often gets 'stuck in the gullet'.

Stomach

Surprisingly little has been written about the stomach in Sjögrens. In theory, abnormalities of the protective 'mucous membrane' in the stomach in Sjögrens might render the stomach more prone to damage from drugs such as anti-inflammatories. There are a few case reports suggesting that the volume of acid secretion in the stomach is quite low and in a few patients no gastric secretion (achlorhydria) was also reported. In practice, this does not appear to have proved a common problem.

G. Hughes et al., *Sjögren's Syndrome in Clinical Practice*,
DOI 10.1007/978-3-319-06059-0_6,
© Springer International Publishing Switzerland 2014

Small and Large Bowel

Again, Sjögren's syndrome seems to cause few major bowel problems. However, some of the diseases often associated with Sjögren's syndrome, can and do cause bowel symptoms – some of these are listed:

Coeliac Disease

Coeliac disease, another of the auto-immune disorders, is associated with Sjögren's syndrome.

The condition is known to be due to sensitivity to gluten – a constituent of wheat products. In severe cases (e.g.: in children before the cause became recognised), the flatulence, abdominal pain, diarrhoea and malabsorption, often lead to severe weight loss and vitamin deficiencies. Nowadays, with strict avoidance of gluten-containing food products (lists of which are obtainable in most chemists), Coeliac patients can lead a normal life. In the past few decades, it has become clear that 'milder' forms of Coeliac disease are common – sometimes with negative Coeliac antibody tests. In any Sjögrens patients with 'food intolerance', this diagnosis is worth considering and a trial of gluten avoidance.

Other 'Food Allergies'

A history of food intolerance is common in Sjögrens. Whether the symptoms are secondary to an allergy or down to other mechanisms is unclear.

In our clinic we certainly find that a number of Sjögren's patients do have strong histories of food intolerance. Although there are no widely accepted tests for the problem, other than 'trial and error', it is always worth the patient keeping a working diary in order to detect any recurring patterns, e.g.: Some years ago we published the case of a doctor's wife who had Sjögrens, with rapidly worsening arthritis. At that time we were researching into aspects of food intolerance.

We found that this patient had demonstrable antibodies to the cheese protein Casein, and this doctor's wife loved cheese! Within months of a diary free diet, the arthritis had totally abated.

Low Thyroid

As has been mentioned, it is not uncommon to find a 'lazy' thyroid in some Sjögrens patients. The common symptoms of 'hypothyroidism' are cold intolerance, mental and physical sluggishness, 'pins and needles' in the hands, (carpal tunnel syndrome) – and constipation. Thus, in a Sjögrens patient developing worsening constipation, one line of enquiry is to test the thyroid.

Hughes Syndrome

Also frequently overlapping with Sjögren's is Hughes Syndrome (Antiphospholipid Syndrome/APS). This condition – 'sticky blood' – can cause impaired circulation to the limbs, as well as to internal organs such as the brain, e.g.; (migraine) and heart (angina). Another organ which can be starved of a full blood supply in Hughes Syndrome, is the gut (Fig. 6.1). After a large meal, the jumped-into-action gut requires an increased blood supply. As with the heart, if adequate oxygen is not forthcoming, there is pain in the so called 'abdominal angina' – classically coming on an hour or so after a big meal.

Pancreas

The pancreas is a major digestive organ. Failure of the pancreas can result in malabsorption, with pale, fatty stools, diarrhoea and, ultimately signs and symptoms of malnutrition and vitamin deficiency. Although the structure of the pancreas has a number of similarities to the parotid gland.

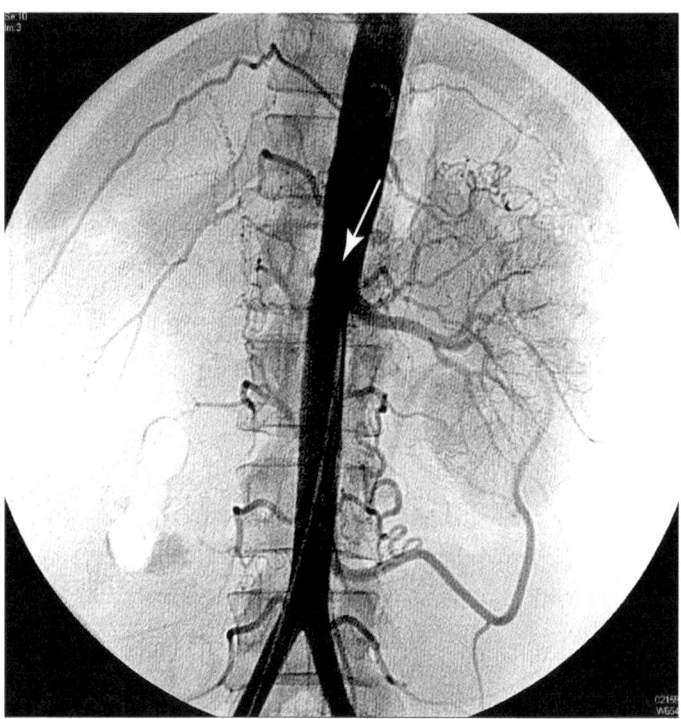

FIGURE 6.1 A digital subtraction angiogram of abdominal aorta shows completely occluded coeliac trunk in a patient with Hughes syndrome

Chapter 7
Bladder, Vagina, Kidney

Bladder

Bladder problems are common (and almost certainly under-recognised) in Sjögrens patients. Common complaints are of urinary frequency, stinging on passing urine and lower abdominal discomfort.

Urine samples, sent to exclude urinary infections are generally clear of bacteria, usually showing a few red and white blood cells only.

The probable reason for the symptoms is, once again, the imperfect mucous membrane lining of a bladder and the bladder exit, the urethra. Very occasionally the condition worsens into a condition known as 'interstitial cystitis' a chronic condition of the bladder wall – a condition which requires expert urological care.

Vagina

Similarly, the vaginal wall can become dry, leading to discomfort on intercourse. Another problem arising from the imperfect vaginal wall is a predilection to develop vaginal thrush. Interestingly, a number of years ago, we found that many our Sjögren's patients and lupus patients had abnormal cervical smear tests. They never turned out to be malignant, but nevertheless, caused considerable anxiety.

G. Hughes et al., *Sjögren's Syndrome in Clinical Practice*,
DOI 10.1007/978-3-319-06059-0_7,
© Springer International Publishing Switzerland 2014

Our theory for this finding is that the abnormal cervical smear reflects the abnormal dry local environment in the vagina in some of these patients.

Kidney

The dryness in the bladder fortunately doesn't appear to result in an increased risk of kidney infections. However, the kidney can occasionally, be directly involved in Sjögrens – a figure usually put at around 5 %, though we believe the figure to be lower. As with other organs, the Sjögrens pathology is one of organ infiltration by lymphocytes.

Unlike lupus, where kidney disease can be life threatening, in Sjögrens the effects are usually milder. Interestingly, the parts of the kidney more affected in Sjögrens are the filtering tubules (tubulointerstitial nephritis), rather than the filters themselves (the so-called glomeruli). The kidney tubules are more than mere drainage pipes. They play an important part in regulating the acid/alkali milieu, as well as the body's level of elements such as potassium and chlorine.

Two well known, though relatively uncommon consequences of kidney tubule malfunction in Sjögrens are low potassium, and so called 'renal tubular acidosis'. The leaking of potassium into the urine can lead to a low level in the blood – leading in turn to muscle weakness! Thus measurement of serum potassium level is an important investigation of Sjögrens. Along with potassium, bicarbonates are, sometimes excessively, lost through the urine retaining hydrogen ions in the body which results in an acidosis (renal tubular acidosis).

Acute or chronic tubulointerstitial nephritis with defects in tubular function is the predominant lesion in biopsy-proven renal involvement. Distal (type I) renal tubular acidosis is the most common clinical finding, leading to mild symptoms but also to potentially life-threatening complications, such as hypokalemic (low potassium) paralysis (Fig. 7.1).

Renal tubular acidosis can lead to kidney stones, and, in severe cases calcification of the kidney itself ('nephrocalcinosis') (Fig. 7.2).

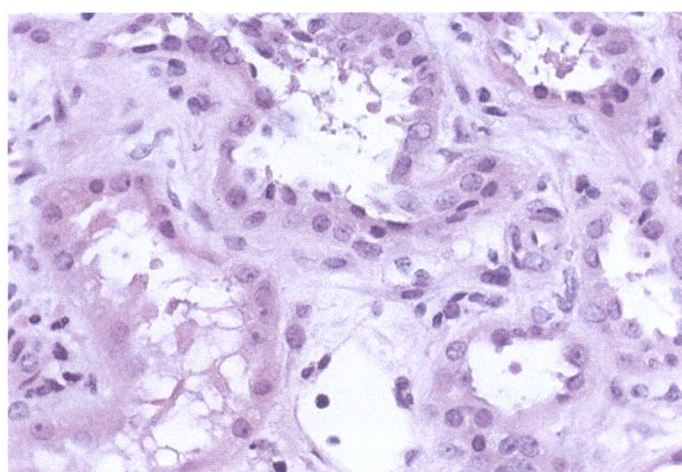

FIGURE 7.1 A renal biopsy showing renal tubular damage due to intestitial nephritis in a patient with Sjögren's syndrome

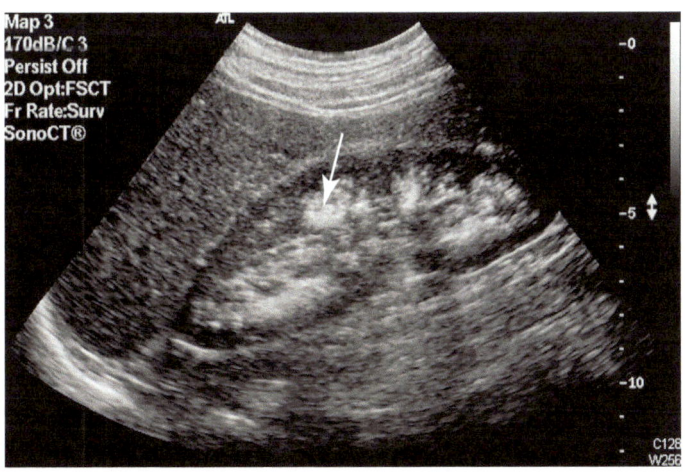

FIGURE 7.2 A renal ultrasound showing nephrocalcinosis (calcium deposits in the kidney - white areas - see *arrow*) in a patient with Sjögren's syndrome who had renal tubular acidosis

Therapy

Corticosteroids often help at early stages with good results. Immunosuppressive therapy such as mycophenolate mofetil, azathioprine, belimumab and rituximab have shown improvement on long term follow up. Similarly hypokalemia and low bicarbonates replacement are also essential part of therapy. It should, however, be stressed that serious kidney problems are rare in most Sjögren's studies.

Chapter 8
The Nervous System

Traditionally, the nervous system is divided into two parts – the central nervous system (brain and spinal cord) and the 'peripheral' nervous system (the nerves, or wiring system).

Brain and Spinal Cord

Cerebral and spinal problems are unusual in Sjögrens. Although in previous decades, a number of reports of stroke, and of multiple sclerosis-like features were reported, the true nature of these associations remains unclear. The manifestations depend on the part of the brain/spinal cord involved. This may present as stroke, seizures, movement disorders, meningoencephalitis or inflammation of the spinal cord (transverse myelitis). Occasionally patients may present with mood disorders such as depression and other behavioural problems. The discovery of the antiphospholipid/Hughes syndrome, and its overlap with Sjögrens (see Chap. 11), has changed our views on the subject. Time will tell, but it seems clear to us that some cases of stroke or MS-like disorders in Sjögrens may be due more to 'sticky blood' (Hughes syndrome) than to Sjögrens itself.

G. Hughes et al., *Sjögren's Syndrome in Clinical Practice*,
DOI 10.1007/978-3-319-06059-0_8,
© Springer International Publishing Switzerland 2014

Trigeminal Neuralgia

This common condition crops up frequently in Sjögrens. The trigeminal ('three branches') nerve arises in front of the ear and supplies one half of the face. The top branch supplies the forehead, the middle branch, the cheek and side of the nose and the lower branch the jaw. Trigeminal neuralgia (uncomfortable, sometimes marked, nerve pain and changed sensation), thus can affect the whole side of the face, or only one part (e.g.: involvement of the lower branch is often put down to toothache).

A variety of treatments are available, including ultrasound, and medications such as Tegretol (carbamazepin), gabapentin, or pregabalin.

Other Cranial Nerves

The head and neck are supplied by 12 pairs of cranial nerves. A number of reports of cranial nerve lesions have been reported in Sjögrens, leading to a variety of outcomes such as double vision and facial weakness. They are rare.

Peripheral Neuropathy

Numbness and tingling and symptoms such as burning in the feet is an occasional complication of Sjögrens. Patients may have difficulty in balancing due to loss of position sense (ataxia). Reflexes may be absent. Some patients present with progressive weakness in the limbs (mononeuritis multiplex) and/or radiculopathy with symptoms similar to disc prolapse (sciatica). Nerve tests in such cases may reveal impaired 'nerve conduction' (faulty electrics). However, as discussed on page 22, peripheral neuropathy can also result from an impaired blood supply secondary to purpura affecting the lower leg.

One recent study reported the presence of low vitamin D levels in patients with Sjögrens with peripheral neuropathy.

Autonomic Neuropathy

The autonomic part of the nervous system controls the opening and contraction of blood vessels, secretion by glands and some aspects of bowel and bladder function. The secretory function of glands depends on the sympathetic and parasympathetic innervation of the autonomic nervous system. Failure of the parasympathetic nervous system can result in sicca (dryness) syndrome, the cardinal feature of Sjögren's syndrome. Fatigue seen in Sjögren's syndrome is sometimes also attributed to autonomic dysfunction. It may present as postural hypotension (drop in blood pressure on standing) resulting in to giddiness. Abnormalities of this rather mysterious nerve network have been described both in Sjögrens and in Hughes Syndrome.

Chapter 9
Joints, Tendons, Muscles

Introduction

Next to fatigue, aches and pains are the commonest complaints in Sjögren's Syndrome. The symptoms include stiffness, muscle pain, joint pain and even tendon pain – often so diffuse that it is hard for the patient to be specific about the exact sites of the symptoms. Not surprisingly, many patients are diagnosed at some stage as having 'fibromyalgia'. One of the clinical hallmarks of the symptoms in Sjögrens is the wide fluctuation seen in severity over a period of time. In some younger patients, the symptoms are worse in the few days before periods (in a number of cases, we have resorted to using stronger drugs such as low dose steroids just for those few pre-menstrual days in order to keep the patient 'on the road').

Joints

The 'pattern' of joint involvement is important to physicians dealing with rheumatic disease. In Sjögrens, as in rheumatoid arthritis, the pattern is usually symmetrical, affecting left and right equally, and affecting small joints such as the knuckles, wrists, toes prominently. Usually, there is a little actual swelling, but the joints are tender to touch (e.g.: heavy handshake). One of the characteristics of the arthritis of Sjögrens is its variability. Patients can, for example, suffer from periods of arthritis for many months and then the symptoms inexplicably subside.

G. Hughes et al., *Sjögren's Syndrome in Clinical Practice*,
DOI 10.1007/978-3-319-06059-0_9,
© Springer International Publishing Switzerland 2014

Sjögren's and Rheumatoid Arthritis

Up to 30 % of patients with rheumatoid arthritis have accompanying Sjögrens. Such patients are diagnosed with 'secondary' Sjögrens, as opposed to 'primary' Sjögren's, a condition with dryness and enlarged glands, but without accompanying rheumatoid arthritis or other connective tissue disease. Having said this, it can be difficult for the physician or the patient suffering from widespread joint pains to know whether this will remain as Sjögren's, or develop into joint -damaging rheumatoid arthritis. There are some helpful tips. Firstly, joint erosion ('a mouse nibbling at the cheese') is a feature of active rheumatoid rather than Sjögren's. Secondly, blood tests can be of some help. Anti-Ro (see Chap. 14) is more closely linked with Sjögrens, while the important new blood test 'anti-CCP' is more predictive of the development of rheumatoid arthritis.

Some years ago a consensus of 'classification criteria' for Sjögren's syndrome was drawn up. This will be discussed in Chap. 14.

Tendons

In lupus, it is notable that tendons are often more predominantly involved than joints. Thus some patients cannot fully straighten their fingers, while others develop 'hitch-hiking thumbs'. Larger tendons such as wrist, ankle and Achilles may be involved. The same is true (though usually to a far lesser degree) in Sjögrens.

Usually the attack of 'tendonitis' in short lived, though in some cases, more chronic involvement can lead to tendon rupture or to shortening and slight deformity (Fig. 9.1).

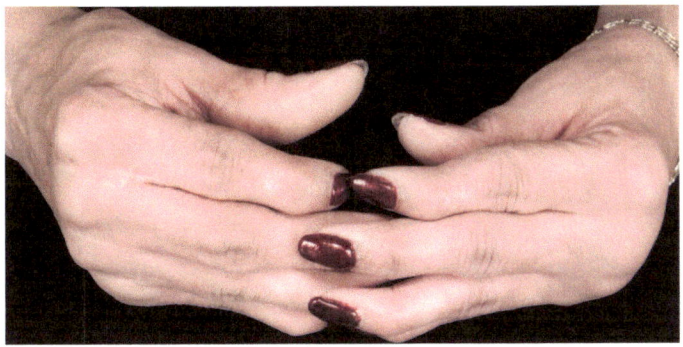

FIGURE 9.1 Shortening of tendons (Jaccoud's arthropathy) seen in a patient with Sjögren's syndrome

Muscles

Muscle aches are also common in Sjögrens. There may be tenderness, though weakness is not usually a prominent feature. Tests for muscle inflammation such as the blood test called CK or CPK (creatine phospho-kinase) are usually normal. Rarely however, true myositis, an autoimmune condition of muscle, can accompany Sjögrens. Here, usually the picture is very different, with muscle wasting, weight loss and marked weakness (e.g.; getting up from a low chair). The muscle electric test (electromyogram (EMG)) then shows intense activity. The MRI may show inflamed areas in the muscle groups (Figs. 9.2 and 9.3), and the CK/CPK level may be in the thousands. (a rare association with Sjögren's it should be said). A more modest form of 'low-grade' myositis with muscle aches, a moderately raised CPK and minor changes in the EMG is sometimes seen.

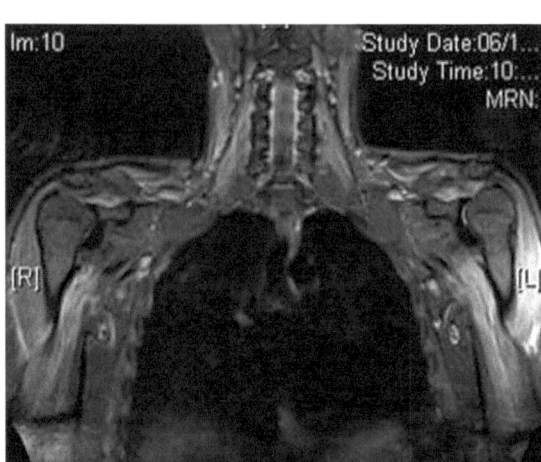

FIGURE 9.2 Magnetic resonance imaging showing myositis in a patient with Sjögren's syndrome (bright signals in shoulder and neck muscles)

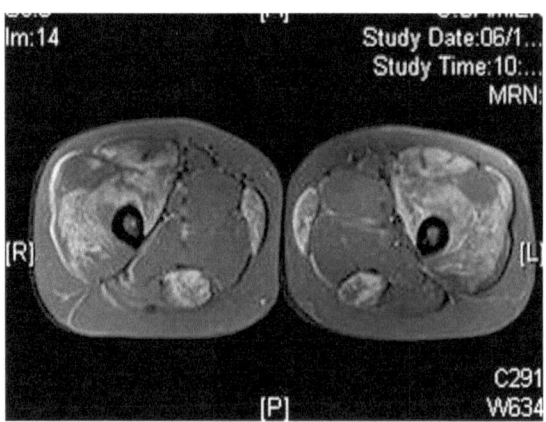

FIGURE 9.3 Magnetic resonance imaging showing myositis in a patient with Sjögren's syndrome (bright signal indicates muscle inflammation)

Chapter 10
Sjögren's and Lymphoma

Introduction

There is an increased incidence of lymphoma in Sjögrens. While this is often the first thing a patient reads on an internet search, there are important figures and facts to note. Firstly, the tendency to lymphoma is almost always confined to patients with primary Sjögrens, and not the larger group of patients with conditions such as rheumatoid arthritis and 'secondary' Sjögrens. Secondly, the group of patients most at risk are those with:

- Persistently enlarged salivary glands (for example; very big parotids).
- Persistently enlarged lymph nodes and spleen.
- Recurrent purpura.
- Peripheral neuropathy

In addition, the blood tests can be helpful: lymphoma is more common in those with positive anti Ro/La antibodies, persistent low complement C3 and C4 levels, lymphopenia or with mixed cryoglobulinaemia (see Chap. 11).

G. Hughes et al., *Sjögren's Syndrome in Clinical Practice*,
DOI 10.1007/978-3-319-06059-0_10,
© Springer International Publishing Switzerland 2014

Features of Lymphoma (Figs. 10.1 and 10.2)

The lymphomas (tumours of the lymphoid system) are known to arise from B cells (a type of white cell involved in the process of antibody production) – so called Non-Hodgkins lymphoma (NHL). While most arise in the salivary glands, others can arise in the pharynx, stomach or liver. Widespread lymph node enlargement is common. Perhaps surprisingly, many of these lymphomas remain localised for years, and for most patients, treatment is successful.

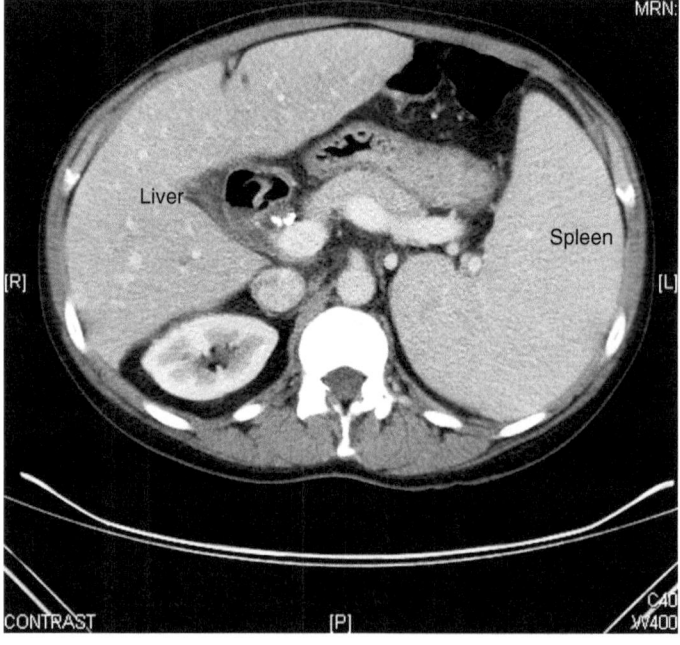

FIGURE 10.1 A CT scan of the abdomen showing enlarged liver and spleen in a patient with non-Hodgkins lymphoma

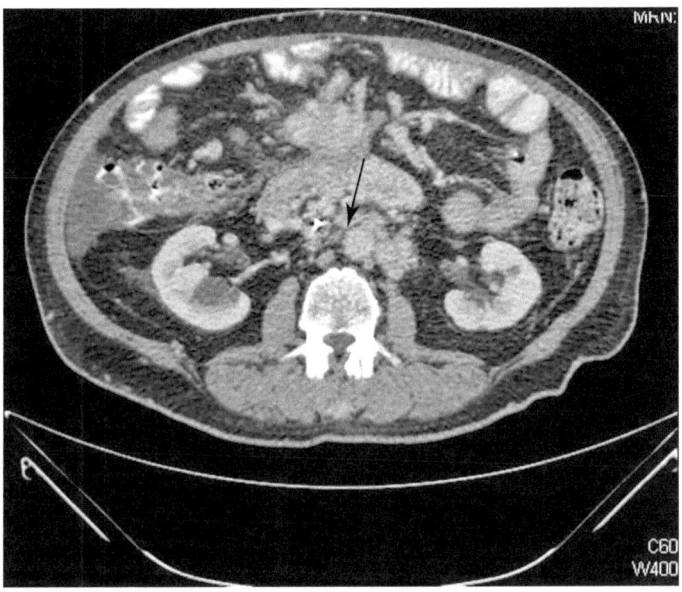

FIGURE 10.2 A Ct scan abdomen showing enlarged para-aortic lymph nodes (*arrowed*) in a patient with non-Hodgkins lymphoma

Relationship Between Lymphoma, Sjögrens, Lupus and Vitamin D

B cell lymphomas have been known to be associated with some 'B cell' autoimmune diseases for many years. The prevalence of NHL in Sjögrens is put at 4 %, with a time interval between Sjögrens diagnosis and lymphoma development of 7½ years.

It should be stressed that the complication is strongly associated with some of the features listed above and careful diagnosis is important, e.g.; this malignancy (notably lymphoma) was once reported as being more common in lupus. Certainly not the case in our own experience – a look at the lupus literature citing lymphoma risk includes many patients in their 50s and 60s. This is more likely to be primary Sjögrens. Just to add to the discussion, lymphoma has been seen in a number of first degree relatives of our auto-immune patients (further discussion in Chap. 16).

Chapter 11
Sjögren's Overlaps

Sjögren's and Allergy

Many patients aged, say, 50, give a history of lifelong allergies – skin allergies, mild asthma, food allergies. Common in the past was an allergy to Septrin – an antibiotic often used for urine infections – in some cases this allergy was severe – life threatening – with damage to internal organs, severe mucosal ulceration ('Stevens-Johnson Syndrome') and other features. In the days when gold salts were used to treat rheumatoid arthritis, skin rashes were common – especially so in those RA patients with associated Sjögrens (Fig. 11.1).

Sjögren's and Hughes Syndrome

We have not yet formally carried out a proper study of the link between Hughes Syndrome and Sjögrens. However, in a busy clinical practice with 1,200 cases of Hughes Syndrome (Antiphospholipid Syndrome) on our 'books', we estimate that between 30 and 50 % have some features of Sjögrens, even if only a dry Schirmer's tear test. Clearly, the link is extremely important, both in diagnosis and treatment. Sjögrens can account for some of the symptoms seen in Hughes Syndrome – fatigue, aches and pains – while Hughes Syndrome can, in turn, have been responsible for some reported features of Sjögren's – neurological lesions, for example (Fig. 11.2).

G. Hughes et al., *Sjögren's Syndrome in Clinical Practice*,
DOI 10.1007/978-3-319-06059-0_11,
© Springer International Publishing Switzerland 2014

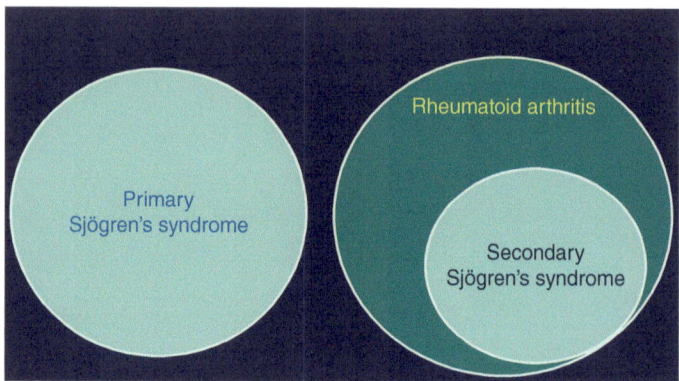

FIGURE 11.1 Primary and secondary Sjögren's syndrome is associated with another condition, usually rheumatoid arthritis

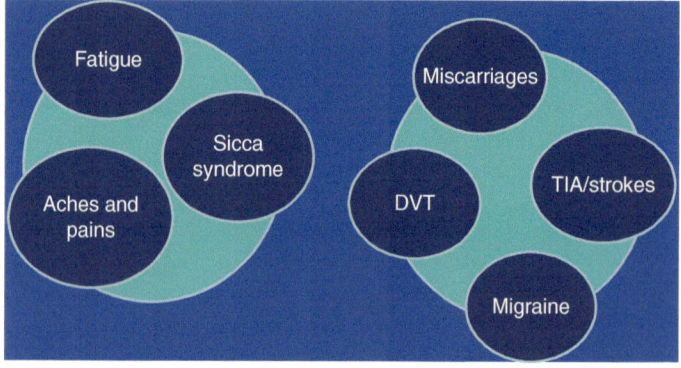

FIGURE 11.2 Salient features of Sjogren's syndrome (on the left) and Hughes syndrome (on the right)

Sjögrens and Thyroid Disease

The same is true of thyroid disease, especially hypo-thyroidism and Hashimoto's disease (autoimmune thyroid disease). Some studies have put the prevalence of thyroid diseases at up to one third of all Sjögrens patients.

In clinical practice, asking the question of a Hughes Syndrome patients, e.g.: "Is there anyone in your family with thyroid problems?"

"Yes – my sister, one aunt and two cousins". All will almost certainly have features of Sjögrens Syndrome.

The links between Sjögrens, Hughes Syndrome and hypo-thyroidism are so strong that we have taken to calling these conditions 'The big three'.

Sjögrens and Lupus

In so many ways, lupus and Sjögrens are cousins, but with different faces:

Lupus – 15–40 year olds. Danger of kidney disease.
Sjögrens – 30–60 year olds – not life threatening.

The other link is timing: It is common to see patients who, in their 20s had active lupus, gradually settle down, and who, on annual clinic follow-up, are left in their 50s or 60s with residual Sjögrens – occasional aches and pains, dry eyes, fatigue, but no longer life threatening. In this example, we are talking about secondary Sjögrens. It must be stressed that primary Sjögrens and lupus are quite different beasts – both in clinical features, in age groups, in blood tests – and in their clinical course.

Sjögren's, Pregnancy, and Newborn (Anti Ro (SSA) and La (SSB) Antibodies)

Anti Ro and anti La antibodies can cross the placental barrier. Transplacental transfer of these antibodies occurs in preg-nancy. This may result in a transient skin rash "neonatal lupus" and haematological changes in the new born or a in permanent congenital heart block.

The typical cutaneous manifestations include erythema-tous, scaly, annular lesions on the face, with slight central atrophy and photosensitivy, clinically and histologically simi-lar to subacute cutaneous lupus ("neonatal lupus" [Fig. 11.3]). These lesions may occur at birth or after exposure to the sun.

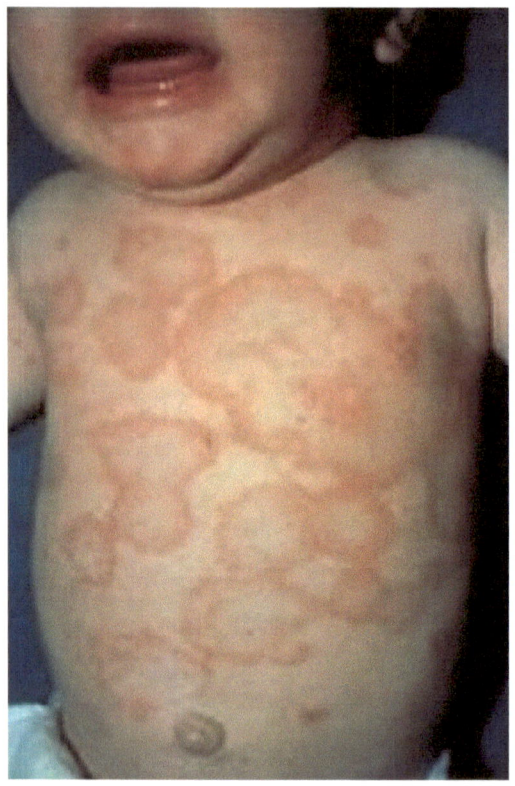

FIGURE 11.3 Neonatal lupus rash in a new born with mother having positive Ro antibodies

Generally the long term outcome is good and these rashes disappear after about 6 months without leaving any residual scars.

The permanent damage to the heart is much more serious complication. These antibodies can attach the conducting system in the heart causing inflammation, fibrosis and scarring. This is a rare complication occurring about 2 % of patients carrying anti Ro or anti La antibodies. However a mother whose 1st child has congenital heart block (CHB) (Fig. 11.4), the chances of 2nd child with CHB increases

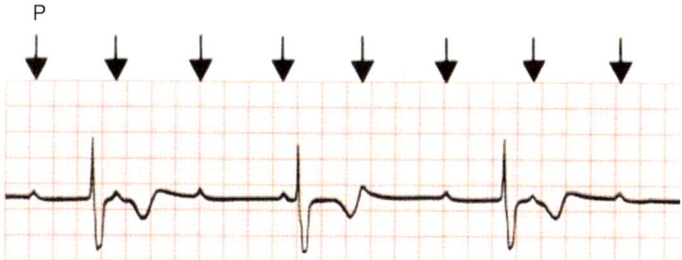

FIGURE 11.4 Congenital heart block in a new born with mother having positive Ro antibodies

almost to one in five. The end result is congenital heart block of varying severity. It is not uncommon to see 1st degree and 2nd degree heart block vary in severity but 3rd degree heart block is irreversible. It is advisable to have a regular echocardiogram for the foetus where mothers are known to have positive antibodies.

Sjögrens and Cryoglobulinemia

This manifestation of Sjögrens presents as a purpuric rash on the legs and occasionally with involvement of kidneys. First sign of renal involvement is protein leak in the urine which can be measured by dipstick.

Sjögrens and Fibromyalgia

Fibromyalgia is a symptom complex, with aches and pains, stiffness and fatigue. Clinically, a feature is local tenderness at a number of sites such as around the shoulder blades. There are no specific blood tests and treatment in largely empirical, with anti-inflammatories, anti-depressives and sleep medicines to the fore. Clearly, with such a nebulous collection of features and no firm defining markers, prevalence varies enormously. A number of patients with other conditions such as lupus, rheumatoid and polymyalgia come under the differential diagnosis, but perhaps most commonly, Sjögrens patients travel the 'fibromyalgic' route on the way to diagnosis. At the present time, there are few good data on the overlap between fibromyalgia and other rheumatological and autoimmune conditions. About 1 in 20 people with rheumatoid arthritis, lupus or Sjögren's syndrome have fibromyalgic symptoms.

Chapter 12
General Treatment

Introduction

Sjögrens Syndrome can be an up and down illness. Treatment therefore must be tailored closely to the patient's symptoms. For many patients, no drug therapy is required – for others short term courses of treatment may suffice. During flares, steroids may be needed. One of the first rules of treatment is to be alert to 'non-Sjögrens symptoms which may be lurking. Underlying thyroid problems will respond to thyroid replacement – (thyroxine – remember this is not a 'drug', but rather a natural replacement for an underperforming thyroid gland). Hughes syndrome must be looked for. Features of this illness such as headaches, memory problems, balance problems, often show a marked response to as little as one 'baby' aspirin (75–100 mg) a day – though of course others may require more substantial anticoagulation. A check on vitamin D level is also advised. It is interesting to find that many patients with lupus and with Sjögrens have low vitamin D levels (the accepted normal level is above 75 units). Important, because vitamin D is not just for bones, but is now known to be required for a healthy immune response.

G. Hughes et al., *Sjögren's Syndrome in Clinical Practice*,
DOI 10.1007/978-3-319-06059-0_12,
© Springer International Publishing Switzerland 2014

Diet

Sjögrens does seem to be a condition in which food 'allergies' (or food intolerances) are common. Sensitivity to wheat has already been mentioned, but many patients give clear histories of intolerance to other foods and drinks.

Unfortunately, 'food allergy' is not an exact science, and there is a real danger of spending hard earned money in clinics promising success. Our initial advice is to use your own best judgement – to keep a mental (or written) diary of times when the symptoms seem more troublesome. Is there a pattern emerging of links to certain foods?

Eyes

Impaired tear coverage in the eyes can lead to damage to the conjunctiva and even the cornea. 'Artificial tears' are very valuable in preventing these complications. A variety of these are available from chemists, most based on cellulose, which has similar properties to natural tears. Importantly, most avoid the use of chemical preservatives. The drops can be used as frequently as the individual wishes – hourly if necessary. If they are used very often, however, it is vital to use 'preservative-free' drops as the preservative itself can irritate the eyes if used very frequently. The choice of artificial tears depends on the individual – some prefer 'runny' products such as 'hypromellose' while others prefer more viscous preparations such as 'viscotears' or 'celluvisc (Fig. 12.1)'.

Other measures include avoidance, where possible, of prolonged exposure to low humidity (e.g.: strong air conditioning), and, if at all possible, of higher doses of drugs which can cause eye dryness, e.g.; diuretics, some anti-hypertensives, and anti-depressants such as amytriptyline, (itself a drug widely used to treat fibromyalgia – a diagnosis many Sjögrens patients know well). Rarely, in severe cases, ophthalmologists may plug the draining tear ducts in the lower

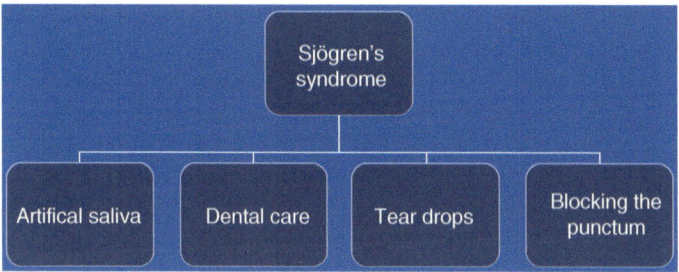

FIGURE 12.1 Treatment of sicca syndrome

(and sometimes also upper) eyelids in order to allow a longer duration of the tears on the cornea. If this works the ducts can be permanently blocked by cauterisation.

Mouth

Unfortunately, treatment of the dry mouth of Sjögrens is often less successful than that of the dry eye. Some find the sucking of sugar-free lozenges, or the use of sugar free gum helpful in stimulating saliva secretion. The lack of saliva makes the teeth more susceptible to damage from sugar, so sugary foods, sweets and drinks should be avoided. Most patients carry small bottles of water with them, and many take a jug of water to bed. Commercial preparations of 'artificial saliva' sprays can sometimes be helpful. Gels such as bioxtra or biotene can be helpful. Patients are advised to brush their teeth after meals, floss at least once a day and use a diluted alcohol-free fluoride or chlorhexidine mouthwash. A toothpaste with high fluoride content can help protect the teeth.

A number of drugs have been tried. One which is widely used is pilocarpine (Salagen), 5 mg three times a day. Unfortunately, this dosage frequently produces unacceptable side effects, notably sweating and flushing. Our own practice is to suggest a trial of one tablet a day – or even only on days when the patient is likely to be speaking more than usual (e.g.; in a job interview, where the stress worsens the dryness further). One of the sequelae of the dry mouth is dental caries. Patients are counselled regarding oral hygiene, and good dental care is vital. Many large hospital dental departments now run special Sjögrens clinics. Rarely, one or other parotid or submandibular glands becomes suddenly swollen and painful. This is often due either to blockage by a stone, or to an acute infection. Both need rapid medical attention.

Lifestyle

Most Sjögrens live a full and active life. Some, sensitive to excess UV light find that they are better avoiding prolonged sun exposure.

Even for those with muscle and joint pains, exercise is allowed – even a small amount of exercise has been shown to reduce fatigue levels, and sensible exercising does <u>not</u> increase joint damage – a question raised by many patients.

Chapter 13
Drug Treatment

Plaquenil (hydroxychloroquine)

This is one of the gentlest, yet most successful medicines in our pharmacy. It is a medicine which has proved helpful in countless numbers of Sjögren's patients (Fig. 13.1).

The chemical name is hydroxychloroquine, which shows us that it comes from the quinine family. Quinine itself is a natural product, coming from the bark of the South American Cinchona tree, widely used by the natives for its medicinal properties, probably for centuries.

In 1886, Dr. Payne, a Consultant at St Thomas' Hospital in London, published a paper suggesting that quinine might also be useful in lupus, especially for joint pains and fatigue.

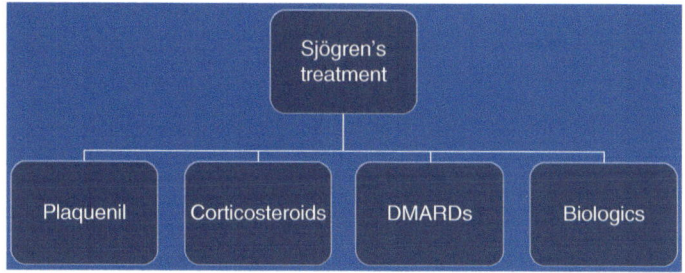

FIGURE 13.1 Various modalities of drug therapy in Sjögren's syndrome

G. Hughes et al., *Sjögren's Syndrome in Clinical Practice*,
DOI 10.1007/978-3-319-06059-0_13,
© Springer International Publishing Switzerland 2014

From quinine, the anti-malarial drug chloroquine was developed, and for decades become one of the mainstays of anti-malaria treatment. Chloroquine also became widely used in the treatment of lupus ….. and of Sjögren's Syndrome. Unfortunately, it was a drug with many side effects, especially nausea. But one side effect overshadowed the rest – retinal toxicity ….. damage to the eye. Sadly, some countries still use chloroquine but, fortunately, most have transferred to <u>hydroxy</u>-chloroquine (trade name Plaquenil), which does not have this toxicity other than in a few exceptionally rare cases.

There are now many large safety studies of Plaquenil, including our own 5 year study, when patients on 5 years of daily Plaquenil showed zero retinal changes. Side effects of Plaquenil are rare – indeed routine blood tests are unnecessary. We routinely use Plaquenil through pregnancy!

For most patients, a dose of 1 tablet (Plaquenil 200 mg) a day is sufficient. The medicine is slow to kick in (3–4 weeks), but when it does, most patients notice the definite improvement in energy. In the past some physicians advocated a 'loading dose', e.g.; 3 tablets a day, but we avoid this as this high dose can cause a loose tummy. More important, and worryingly for the patient, a high dose can also cause slight difficulties in focusing. These do not result in eye damage, and are reversible on returning to the normal dose of one a day – but the effect on patient confidence can be disastrous. Plaquenil is now used around the world, both for mild lupus and for Sjögrens. In the main benefits are in the symptoms of fatigue and aches and pains, though some patients definitely show improvement in tear and saliva secretion.

Benefits and Drawbacks of Plaquenil

Benefits

Improves fatigue
Improves aches and pains
Slight improvement in tear and saliva secretion

Anti-clotting (slight)
Photo-protective (very useful against sun rashes)
Lowers cholesterol (slight)

Problems

Mild (not effective in severe arthritis)
Allergy (rare)
'Gassy Stomach' (usually in doses of 2 or 3 a day)
Slight skin pigmentation (skin moles become darker)

Many patients remain on Plaquenil for years, as background 'preventative' medicine while others vary the dose – e.g.; from as little as three tablets a week increasing to 1½ or 2 a day during flares.

Mepacrine (Also Called Quinacrine)

This drug is also part of the quinine family. It is particularly effective in some cases of skin lupus, and is a second choice if, for any reason, plaquenil is insufficient. It does, however, have problems. It is bitter, and, in fair skinned patients, causes yellowish pigmentation of the skin after some months. Its use is therefore limited.

One useful practice is to add low dose mepacrine (e.g.; 1 tablet of 100 mg 3 times a week) to the usual 1 Plaquenil a day, in patients where the skin improvement is unsatisfactory. It has little place in Sjögrens.

Disease Modifying Agents – DMARDs

Steroids

Steroids have a limited use in Sjögrens. Ideally, they should not be used for the long term treatment of Sjögrens, but are very valuable in short-term crisis or flare ups. The commonly used steroid is called Prednisolone, and comes in 3 strengths – 5, 2.5 and 1 mg. Ideally, doses below 7.5 mg/day daily are the rule.

The most common use of steroids in Sjögrens is in the management of acute flares – e.g.; of arthritis (or, rarely, of pleurisy). As mentioned earlier, some younger patients with Sjögrens complain of monthly pre-menstrual flares. In such cases, a short course (e.g.: 3–5 days of Prednisolone at a dose of 5–7.5 mg daily is useful).

In the older (e.g.; over 50 years old) Sjögrens patients, the risks of steroids are greater – in particular those from bone-softening (osteoporosis). Most physicians add in a calcium and vitamin D tablet in this group of patients on steroids, in order to protect against osteoporosis.

Azathioprine

This is one of the oldest of the so-called 'immunosuppressive' drugs. Over the years, its position in medicine has been that of a 'steroid-sparing' agent – e.g.; when a patient attempting to reduce steroids fails to get below, say, 10 mg of Prednisolone a day. Some patients cannot tolerate the drug due to nausea, in which case the drug should be withdrawn. On the other hand, azathioprine is safe in pregnancy – important in younger patients with troublesome disease.

Cyclophosphamide

This, is a much stronger immunosuppressive, proved life-saving in severe cases, such as aggressive lupus, or widespread vasculitis. It was particularly successful in the management of lupus nephritis. However, in most cases of Sjögrens, this drug is not indicated, the side effects (low blood counts, cystitis) are too severe for it to be considered in treatment except in rare patients with vasculitis, progressive neuropathy, kidney, lung or skin disease. A prolonged use of oral cyclophospha-mide or high dose intra venous infusions of this drug may lead to infertility in men and premature menopause in women as well as troublesome cystitis (the later protected by the use of a drug called Mesna)

Methotrexate

This drug is used worldwide in the treatment of rheumatoid arthritis, and is extremely effective. It is even used in children with juvenile arthritis (Stills disease), with great effect. Its side effects – liver toxicity in some cases leads to its withdrawal, and a lowering of the blood count in others – are unusual, but do limit the more widespread use of the drug. In Sjögrens, methotrexate is usually reserved for those with prominent or severe arthritis.

Mycophenolate Mofetil

In recent years, this drug has become widely used as an immune-suppressive in lupus, largely taking over from aza-thioprine. It is well tolerated, and has already proved very useful in lupus nephritis. Obviously, experience in the gener-ally milder disease, Sjögrens, is limited. Watch this space. Although well tolerated, this tablet has one major drawback in younger women – it is contra-indicated in pregnancy (unlike azathioprine).

Biologics

This term is used for the new generation of drugs, which have the property of specific 'targeting' of certain cells. They are the 'exocet' missiles of therapy rather than the older 'bombs'. The principle behind these drugs is as follows – a protein 'tar-get' on a particular cell – e.g.; a cancer cell, or, in the case of lupus or Sjögrens, a 'B cell' is identified. An antidote (usually a similar molecule), which then blocks the target is developed.

In auto-immune disease, two major new 'anti-B cell' drugs are now available – rituxumab ('Mabthera') and belimumab ('Benlysta'). Both have proved effective and well tolerated. Both cause a dramatic depletion of the antibody – producing B cells – with very little 'collateral' damage to the other cells. Both drugs are already in use in lupus. Although experience in Sjögrens is limited, recent open label and placebo controlled double blind trials have shown improvement in symptoms such as fatigue, joint pains, cryoglobulinaemia vasculitis, kidney and lung manifestations. There was, however, little improvement in the dryness due to Sjögren's syndrome. It seems reasonable to suggest that both will have a place in the treatment of this B-cell mediated disease. Rituximab is already being used in the routine treatment of patients with Sjögren's syndrome with lymphoma with good benefit.

Chapter 14
Diagnosis I: Blood Tests

Introduction

The clinical history is critical. While many Sjögrens patients don't volunteer a history of dry eyes, eye 'scratchiness or irritation is common. A history of allergies, while not diagnostic, is common, (always ask about septrin allergy). There is often a strong family history of autoimmune disease, especially thyroid (and very especially of the auto-immune condition Hashimoto's thyroiditis). Some years ago, a European collaborative exercise involving 26 cities in 12 countries to a set of validated criteria for the classification of Sjögrens syndrome.

Recently the American College of Rheumatology has proposed an alternative classification criteria for Sjögren's syndrome (Table 14.1).

Antibodies

Blood tests are of value in the diagnosis of Sjögrens, especially if note is taken of the overall picture. Sjögrens patients produce antibodies, and the finding of positive tests for circulating antibodies is one of the hallmarks of the disease. Some are listed here:

'ANA' (anti-nuclear antibodies). Not specific for a particular disease, but raised levels (e.g. over 1 in 80) are commonplace in Sjögrens (and in lupus).

G. Hughes et al., *Sjögren's Syndrome in Clinical Practice*,
DOI 10.1007/978-3-319-06059-0_14,
© Springer International Publishing Switzerland 2014

TABLE 14.1 Proposed classification criteria for Sjögren's syndrome

The classification of SS, which applies to individuals with signs/symptoms that may be suggestive of SS, will be met in patients who have at least two of the following three objective features:

1. Positive serum anti-SSA/Ro and/or anti-SSB/La or (positive rheumatoid factor and ANA titre more than 1:320)

2. Labial salivary gland biopsy exhibiting focal lymphocytic sialadenitis with a focus score equal to or more than 1 focus/4 mm^2

3. Keratoconjunctivitis sicca with ocular staining score 3 (assuming that individual is not currently using daily eye drops for glaucoma and has not had corneal surgery or cosmetic eyelid surgery in the last 5 years)

Prior diagnosis of any of the following conditions would exclude participation in SS studies or therapeutic trials because of overlapping clinical features or interference with criteria tests:

History of head and neck radiation treatment

Hepatitis C infection or acquired immunodeficiency syndrome

Sarcoidosis

Amyloidosis

Graft versus host disease, IgG4-related disease

[Note: Anti DNA antibodies, the hallmark of lupus, are not a feature of Sjögrens. 'Weak positive' lupus DNA result are sometimes reported, but are most often due to technical reasons] Positive ANA tests are found in between 70 and 90 % of Sjögrens patients.

'ENA' This was the name given to a family of antibodies described in the, 1960s ('extractable nuclear antigens'). This mish-mash of antibodies included some which were to prove invaluable in diagnosis. Two were very important in Sjögrens – 'anti Ro and anti La'. (These antibodies also known, for historical reasons as anti SSA and ani SSB). Positive 'anti Ro' and/or 'anti La'antibodies are found in 50–80 % of Sjögrens patients and, when positive, are a useful pointer to the diagnosis.

Other Blood Tests

ESR

This old test, tried and tested, is a guide to inflammation. ESR stands for 'erythrocyte sedimentation rate'.

In simple terms, a thin tube of blood (like a thermometer) is left standing for 1 h. In that time the red cells (erythrocytes) sediment: a few millimetres in healthy individuals, but faster – sometimes over 100 mm – typically when there is inflammation. Thus the 'erythrocyte sedimentation rate' or ESR. Figures of over 50 can be seen in many illnesses, and the ESR has thus become a useful 'screening' test. In Sjögrens patients, the ESR is often raised (e.g.; 30–60) for long periods of time, higher when signs of inflammation such as joint pains are present.

CRP – 'C-Reactive protein'

This rather mysterious protein – found in almost the whole of the animal kingdom, provides another version of the ESR. The CRP level rises in illness – especially in inflammation. In a severe septicaemia, for example, the CRP level can climb into the hundreds. However, rather oddly, in Sjögrens (as well as in lupus), high CRP levels are unusual, unless there is infection. So- it is common in Sjögrens to see, for example, an ESR of 80 and a CRP of zero, a discrepancy which can, in fact, be useful in diagnosis.

Full Blood Count

The normal white cell count is between 4,000 and 10,000 per cu mm. In infections (and on steroids), the white count goes up – and can reach 20,000 or more. In Sjögrens, or the contrary, persistently low white cell counts, known as 'leucopenia' (e.g.; 2,000–3,000 per cu mm) can be a feature.

Again, useful in diagnosis. Perhaps surprisingly, these low white blood counts rarely pose problems such as increased infections.

Anaemia

Mild anaemia is common in Sjögrens. Very occasionally, a more severe anaemia known as 'haemolytic anaemia' is seen – a condition in which circulating antibodies stick to the surface of the red cells, rendering them fragile, and prone to breakdown or 'lysis'.

Rheumatoid Factor

This protein was discovered to be a marker for rheumatoid arthritis and worldwide, became a standard test for this disease. However, rheumatoid factor turned out not to be specific, being found in other situations, notably Sjögrens syndrome, where 50–60 % of patients are positive, despite not having crippling rheumatic disease. Sjogren's syndrome patients do not have positive anti CCP antibodies which are often seen in rheumatoid arthritis.

Cryoglobulins

These are proteins which have the property of coming out of solution in the blood ('precipitating') in the cold and this property can be tested for in the hospital laboratory. They are found in a small number of Sjögrens patients – often those with poor arm and leg circulation. They are usually seen in association with raised levels of blood proteins called 'gamma globulins' – the proteins associated with antibody production (Table 14.2).

TABLE 14.2 Lists the laboratory findings in a large Greek Study

	% of patients
Anaemia	16
Haemolytic anaemia	3
Leukopenia	12
Raised gamma globulins	47
Rheumatoid factor	61
ANA	89
Anti Ro	56
Anti La	30
Cryoglobulins	14

The group of Sjögrens patients with protein variants such as cryoglobulinaemia, 'macroglobulinaemia' and 'paraproteinanaemia' (an abnormal protein seen during protein analysis) are at slightly higher risk of lymphoma (see Chap. 10).

Chapter 15
Diagnosis II: Other Tests

Schirmers Test

Standardised blotting paper strips ('Schirmer papers') are available commercially. The strip is hooked over the lower eyelid for 5 min, and then removed, and the length of 'wet' Schirmer paper recorded (Fig. 2.2). In Sjögrens, it is common to find the paper still completely dry at 5 min, whereas the normal eye often wets the paper in seconds. A result of 5 mm wetting or less in 5 min is considered suggestive of Sjögrens. This test, while seemingly crude, is extremely valuable in clinical practice, especially where there is difficulty in making a firm diagnosis.

Rose Bengal/Lissamine Green Test

This involves a few drops of a dye – 'Rose bengal' (or an alternative – lissamine green) – being placed on the surface of the eye, the surface then being examined by the ophthalmologist with a slit-lamp. The technique is valuable in showing up 'scratches' on what should be a smooth conjunctival surface (Fig. 2.3).

G. Hughes et al., *Sjögren's Syndrome in Clinical Practice*,
DOI 10.1007/978-3-319-06059-0_15,
© Springer International Publishing Switzerland 2014

Scintigraphy

Scanning of the salivary glands using a radioactive maker has been used in the investigation of Sjögrens.

The isotope Technesium 99 is injected intravenously, and the time it takes for the isotope to travel via the blood, through the salivary gland and into the mouth in the saliva measured. In Sjögrens, the process is delayed. The test, though infrequently used, does have a high degree of sensitivity. It requires specialist equipment and expertise and the high doses of radiation means that it is rarely used in practice.

Sialography

This involves the use of a contrast medium to pick up structural changes in the salivary duct system on x-ray. Again, though not widely used, the test (especially using the water soluble media rather than older oil-based agents, which proved very uncomfortable) can be diagnostic in some patients. It is more often used, however, in those few patients with recurrent infections of the salivary glands to rule out a blockage of the parotid duct that could then be unblocked using an expandable tube ('stent').

Lip Biopsy

Biopsy of the salivary glands (parotids and submandibulars) is not practicable. It is traumatic for the patient, and can lead to fistula formation. An advance came with the recognition that perhaps biopsy of the 'minor' salivary glands might be an alternative approach. These small glands, situated in the lower lip can easily feel like 'pinheads' by the tongue. With a small incision under local anaesthetic, a small number of these minor glands can be removed, and studied under the microscope. In Sjögrens, the normal glandular tissue is infiltrated by immune cells (lymphocytes) (Fig. 2.3). For years, this was considered the 'gold standard' for diagnosis. In recent years, this test has been found to be useful in identifying which patients are at greatest risk of lymphoma and, on the other hand, those patients in whom it is unlikely to occur. However, it is unpleasant for the patient, we have largely discontinued using it.

Ultrasound and MRI Scanning

Although not part of the formal classification criteria, ultra-sound scanning of the salivary glands can be very helpful in supporting the diagnosis if a 'swiss-cheese' appearance is seen rather than the bland homogenous appearance of the normal salivary glands. The 'holes' in the 'swiss-cheese' appear to represent areas of inflammation/damage found in Sjögren's syndrome. MRI scanning can also be helpful in patients with enlarged salivary glands, perhaps where they have recently increased in size and there is concern over whether a lymphoma has developed. If a 'lump' is seen within the salivary gland then this requires further investigation with a needle biopsy proceeding to an open biopsy (minor surgery) if a needle biopsy is not diagnostic.

Chapter 16
Causes of Sjögrens

Immunology

Sjögren's syndrome is an "autoimmune disease". It is not clear why some people develop the disease and others escape. It is often seen in people in their 40s or 50s and is much commoner in women. It may present as a single entity or along with other autoimmune diseases such as rheumatoid arthritis or lupus.

Sjögrens is considered a classical auto-immune disease, with lymph cell infiltration of mucous and other secreting glands, and with raised levels of immunoglobulins, providing a range of antibodies. Interestingly, it straddles two groups of auto-immune diseases, the so-called non-organ specific group (such as lupus, where the antibodies are directed against cell (nuclear) materials such as DNA and histones), and the 'organ-specific' group, where antibodies are directed against organs such as the thyroid. Sjögren's patients also frequently give a history of multiple allergies – both to drugs and to foods and colouring agents.

In humans three types of white cells (T cells, B cells and dendritic cells) take part in the immune mechanism. These cells infiltrate the salivary and lachrymal glands and a cascade of chemicals – cytokines (interferon1, interleukins, BAFF) pathways are activated. (There is a strong correlation between raised levels of interferon and anti-Ro and La antibodies seen in Sjögren's syndrome). This leads to inflammation and sometimes destruction of glandular function hence the dry

G. Hughes et al., *Sjögren's Syndrome in Clinical Practice*,
DOI 10.1007/978-3-319-06059-0_16,
© Springer International Publishing Switzerland 2014

mouth and eyes. As the process progresses, the mucosal surfaces become sites of chronic inflammation and the start of a vicious circle. Despite extensive study of the underlying cause of Sjögren's syndrome, the pathogenesis remains obscure. The underlying stimulus for the overactive immune system is still uncertain.

Hormonal

As in the case of its more dangerous cousin lupus, it is clear that hormonal influences play a major role. Both diseases have a high (13:1) female to male ratio. Pre-menstrual flares are common. In the past a number of cases of Sjögrens were reported as worsening when patients were treated with strong oestrogen-containing drugs or injections. Considering the high prevalence in women it is obvious that hormones play a major role in the development of Sjögren's syndrome. Recent reports have suggested the possible lack of male hormones – androgens – in the mechanism of Sjögren's syndrome. It has been observed that the levels of a steroid hormone dehydroepiandrosterone sulphate (DHEA-s) are quite low compared to healthy individuals. It is possible that Sjögren's syndrome patients' low androgen levels may have a direct effect on the target gland.

Viruses

The clinical picture of Sjögrens suggests a possible viral trigger in some cases. One particular virus long under suspicion is the glandular fever virus – the Epstein-Barr or E-B virus. Anecdotally it is very common to obtain a history relating back to this infection. "It all started in my late teens when I went down with glandular fever. I was off school for 2 terms, and never really fully recovered. Lots of my symptoms such as fatigue and 'fibromyalgia' started at that time."

There is anecdotal evidence to suggest the role of E-B virus. For example this virus was detected in the salivary glands of normal people and an exaggerated immune response may cause destruction of the gland; salivary gland biopsies have shown increased levels of E-B virus DNA in Sjögren's patients.

There is a link between genetic signature (HLA DR) in patients' with Sjögren's syndrome and inadequate T cell function. In a case series with Sjögren's syndrome and non-Hodgkin's lymphoma, 1 patient among 14 had E-B virus DNA detected. This finding was similar to those reported in EBV lymphomas occurring in other immunocompromised individuals.

Having said this, there is no proof of a link between EBV and Sjögren's only anecdotal evidence that it might have a role in some patients.

Another virus with Sjögrens-like connections is the hepatitis C virus. This infection, common in certain countries such as Egypt and Italy, can produce chronic lymphoid infiltrate in the salivary glands. The clinical picture does, however, differ from 'classical' Sjögrens in a number of respects, such as the higher frequency of liver involvement in hepatitis C infection. Finally, HIV infection during the AIDS epidemic produced some Sjögrens-like features such as parotid gland swelling and enlarged lymph nodes. However, the resemblances were superficial.

Genetics

The strong family history of auto-immune disease in many Sjögrens patients points towards a genetic predisposition, and not surprisingly genetic studies have turned up a number of associations, e.g.; with the so-called 'histocompatability complex' HLA-DR3. Latest research has shown some links with genes but the presence of abnormal genes does not itself produce Sjögren's syndrome. It is likely that other triggering mechanisms such as infections, or hormones are necessary to supplement the effect of the genes. In Sjögren's syndrome epithelial cells in the glands express high levels of HLA-DR antigens. The glands are infiltrated with CD4+ T cells (white cells) that can produce cytokines, including

IL-2 and interferon-gamma. These cytokines trigger B cell to produce antibodies such as rheumatoid factor. B cells undergo small clonal expansions that can be detected on Southern blot as immunoglobulin gene rearrangements, and SS patients have a markedly increased risk of developing non-Hodgkin's B-cell lymphoma.

Apoptosis and Sjögren syndrome

The mechanism of disposal of dead cells (apoptosis) is also faulty in patients with Sjögren's syndrome. Inability of lymphocytes in the salivary gland to commit to apoptosis, results in prolonged production of inflammatory cytokines and auto-antibodies. Similarly their longer survival may result in the late development of lymphoma in some SS patients.

Environmental Factors

One of the interesting recent 'lessons from nature' has been the 'silicone breast implant' story. Numbers of women who had silicone breast implants (– and particularly those whose implants had ruptured), developed a collection of clinical symptoms. These included fatigue, memory loss, Raynauds, aches and pains and, notably, other features of Sjögrens, including dryness of the eyes and mouth. We now recognise that a number of substances such as silicone (and also, notably, aluminium – contained in a number of vaccines) have the potential to increase the immune response – a property known as 'adjuvants'. Thus aluminium is widely added to certain vaccines to ensure that the recipient's immune response to a certain infection is adequate. In most cases of Sjögrens, clearly, there is no such obvious trigger. Nevertheless, more subtle immune stimulants could well play a part, however minor, in 'stoking the fire', leading to Sjögrens' overactive immune response.

Further Reading Websites

1. British Sjögren's Syndrome Association: http://www.bssa.uk.net/.
2. Sjögren's Syndrome Foundation: http://www.sjogrens.org/.
3. Hughes Syndrome Foundation: www.hughes-syndrome.org.
4. Lupus, UK.
5. Arthritis Research, UK: www.arthritisresearchuk.org.

G. Hughes et al., *Sjögren's Syndrome in Clinical Practice*,
DOI 10.1007/978-3-319-06059-0,
© Springer International Publishing Switzerland 2014

Index

G. Hughes et al., *Sjögren's Syndrome in Clinical Practice*,
DOI 10.1007/978-3-319-06059-0,
© Springer International Publishing Switzerland 2014